Renal Diet

Cookbook

for Beginners

*low-sodium, low-potassium, and
low-phosphorus recipes
for healthy cooking*

By Elizabeth Ross

The information in the following pages is broadly considered a truthful and accurate account of facts and as such, any inattention, use, or misuse of the information in question by the reader will render any resulting actions solely under their purview. There are no scenarios in which the publisher or the original author of this work can be in any fashion deemed liable for any hardship or damages that may befall them after undertaking information described herein.

Additionally, the information in the following pages is intended only for informational purposes and should thus be thought of as universal. As befitting its nature, it is presented without assurance regarding its prolonged validity or interim quality. Trademarks that are mentioned are done without written consent and can in no way be considered an endorsement from the trademark holder.

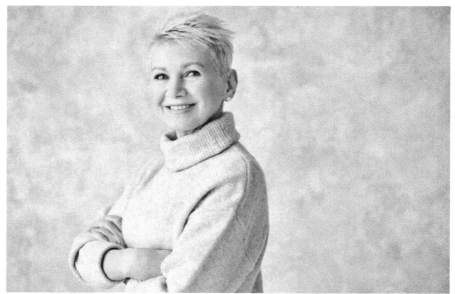

Elizabeth Ross is an American nutritionist born in 1962 in the Hamptons, a seaside resort not far from New York.

She graduated in 1985 in food science and nutrition, thanks to her studies she understands that food is one of the main factors in preventing the worsening of many diseases. For this reason, she decides to devote herself to the improvement of some dietary plans aimed at fighting some diseases.

Her goals are to give the patient a diet based on the patient's problem, guaranteeing stability or even improvement.

She has written many books on specific diets to simplify the disclosure of her food plans and make them accessible to as many people as possible.

Her mission is to make the lives of the people who follow her diets, as simple as possible, giving her in many cases the opportunity to enjoy delicious meals.

Table of content

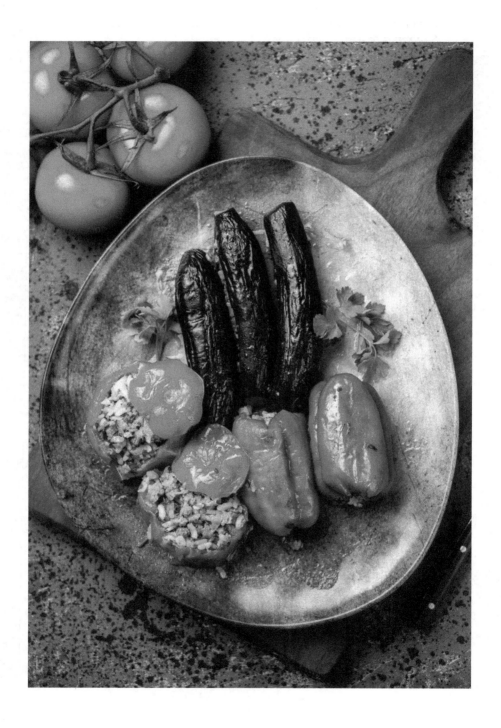

INTRODUCTION

A renal diet is specific to people with kidney issues or disease. Renal diets are high in protein and low in potassium and phosphorus. In addition to a renal diet, you should also avoid foods high in sodium and salt, and you should take a lot of water to help your kidneys function properly.

It's really important to monitor how much protein you're consuming. a lot of protein in the diet can put a strain on the kidneys. It's always best to talk to your doctor about your diet and how to stay healthy. The kidneys helps to remove out the toxins from your body. The diet is one that's low in protein, sodium and potassium. It mostly consists of fresh fruits and vegetables, whole grains and lean meats.

Of course, you should take any prescribed medication your doctor gives you. Whenever you see any of your doctors, make sure they all know every single medication you are using, either prescribed or over the counter, as well as supplements. These can affect your health in more ways than you might realize, and a simple over-the-counter supplement could negatively interact with one of your conditions or medications.

Besides giving your doctor a list of your medications, you should also talk to either your doctor or pharmacist before taking any new over-the-counter medications or supplements. These can cause many problems, which might not be listed on the label. For instance, many painkillers can damage the kidneys and should not be taken by anyone with kidney disease or injury.

Suppose you don't yet have chronic kidney disease, but you or a family member are at risk of developing the condition. In that case, you can reduce your risk and potentially prevent yourself from developing the disease by making healthy lifestyle changes. Remember, you are more likely to develop kidney disease if you have a family history, diabetes, heart disease, or high blood pressure.

By managing the conditions associated with kidney diseases, such as diabetes and high blood pressure, you can benefit your kidney health and the health of your entire body and mind.

You can take to improving your kidney health is managing your blood pressure. Most people only think about the effect blood pressure has on the heart, but it also affects other organs, such as your kidneys. When blood pressure is chronically high, it causes damage to the kidneys. Therefore, you should maintain blood pressure at the goal set by your physician.

When you experience long-term stress, it greatly affects your health. Not only does stress often increase poor life choices, such as smoking, drinking, irregular sleep, and an unhealthy diet. But, chronically high stress increases blood sugar, raises blood pressure, and may lead to depression. You first need to prioritize a healthy lifestyle overall to manage your stress. Exercise, eating well, sleep, and other healthy lifestyle factors can all reduce chronic anxiety. However, you may need different methods of stress relief, as well. Try making a list of any calming activities you find helpful, such as listening to music, meditation, yoga, sketching, reading, or whatever else comes to mind. You can then use this list as inspiration when you are anxious. Whenever you find your stress increased, try completing one or two calming tasks from your list.

As you know, diet is also an important aspect of your lifestyle so you can live better and longer.

Don't forget to do regular doctor check-ups to monitor your progress.

BREAKFAST

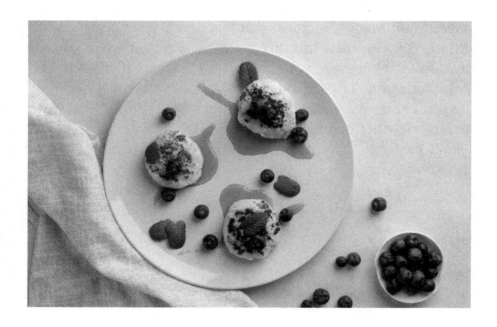

Bulgur, Couscous, and Buckwheat Cereal

Preparation Time: 10 minutes

Cooking Time: 25 minutes

Servings: 4

Ingredients:

- 2 ¼ cups Water
- 1 ¼ cups Vanilla rice milk
- 6 Tbsps. Uncooked bulgur
- 2 Tbsps. Uncooked whole buckwheat
- 1 cup Sliced apple
- 6 Tbsps. Plain uncooked couscous
- ½ tsp. Ground cinnamon

Directions:

1. Heat the water and milk in the saucepan over medium heat. Let it boil.
2. Put the bulgur, buckwheat, and apple.
3. Reduce the heat to low and simmer, occasionally stirring until the bulgur is tender, about 20 to 25 minutes.
4. Remove the saucepan and stir in the couscous and cinnamon—cover for 10 minutes.
5. Put the cereal before serving.

Nutrition: Calories: 159 Fat: 1g Carb: 34g Protein: 4g Sodium: 33mg Potassium: 116m Phosphorus: 130mg

Blueberry Muffins

Preparation Time: 15 minutes

Cooking Time: 30 minutes

Servings: 12

Ingredients:

- 2 cups Unsweetened rice milk
- 1 Tbsp. Apple cider vinegar
- 3 ½ cups All-purpose flour
- 1 cup Granulated sugar
- 1 Tbsp. Baking soda substitute
- 1 tsp. Ground cinnamon
- ½ tsp. Ground nutmeg
- Pinch ground ginger
- ½ cup Canola oil
- 2 Tbsps. Pure vanilla extract
- 2 ½ cups Fresh blueberries

Directions:

1. Preheat the oven to 375F.
2. Prepare a muffin pan and set aside.
3. Stir together the rice milk and vinegar in a small bowl. Set aside for 10 minutes.
4. In a large bowl, stir together the sugar, flour, baking soda, cinnamon, nutmeg, and ginger until well mixed.

5. Add oil and vanilla to the milk and mix.

6. Put milk mixture to dry ingredients and stir well to combine.

7. Put the blueberries and spoon the muffin batter evenly into the cups.

8. Bake the muffins for 25 to 30 minutes or until golden and a toothpick inserted comes out clean.

9. Cool for 15 minutes and serve.

Nutrition: Calories: 331 Fat: 11g Carb: 52g Protein: 6g Sodium: 35mg Potassium: 89mg Phosphorus: 90mg

Buckwheat and Grapefruit Porridge

Preparation Time: 5 minutes

Cooking Time: 20 minutes

Servings: 2

Ingredients:

- ½ cup Buckwheat
- ¼ chopped Grapefruit
- 1 Tbsp. Honey
- 1 ½ cups Almond milk
- 2 cups Water

Directions:

1. Let the water boil on the stove. Add the buckwheat and place the lid on the pan.
2. Lower heat slightly and simmer for 7 to 10 minutes, checking to ensure water does not dry out.
3. When most of the water is absorbed, remove, and set aside for 5 minutes.
4. Drain any excess water from the pan and stir in almond milk, heating through for 5 minutes.
5. Add the honey and grapefruit.
6. Serve.

Nutrition: Calories: 231 Fat: 4g Carb: 43g Protein: 13g Sodium: 135mg Potassium: 370mg Phosphorus: 165mg

Egg and Veggie Muffins

Preparation Time: 15 minutes

Cooking Time: 20 minutes

Servings: 4

Ingredients:

- 4 Eggs
- 2 Tbsp. Unsweetened rice milk
- ½ chopped Sweet onion
- ½ chopped Red bell pepper
- Pinch red pepper flakes
- Pinch ground black pepper

Directions:

1. Preheat the oven to 350F.
2. Spray 4 muffin pans with cooking spray. Set aside.
3. Whisk the milk, eggs, onion, red pepper, parsley, red pepper flakes, and black pepper until mixed.
4. Pour the egg mixture into prepared muffin pans.
5. Bake until the muffins are puffed and golden, about 18 to 20 minutes. Serve.

Nutrition: Calories: 84 Fat: 5g Carb: 3g Protein: 7g Sodium: 75mg Potassium: 117mg Phosphorus: 110mg

Berry Chia with Yogurt

Preparation Time: 35 minutes

Cooking Time: 5 minutes

Servings:4

Ingredients:

- ½ cup chia seeds, dried
- 2 cup Plain yogurt
- 1/3 cup strawberries, chopped
- ¼ cup blackberries
- ¼ cup raspberries
- 4 teaspoons Splenda

Directions:

1. Mix up together Plain yogurt with Splenda, and chia seeds.
2. Transfer the mixture into the serving ramekins (jars) and leave for 35 minutes.
3. After this, add blackberries, raspberries, and strawberries. Mix up the meal well.
4. Serve it immediately or store it in the fridge for up to 2 days.

Nutrition: Calories: 150Fat: 5gCarbs: 19g Protein: 6.8g Sodium: 65mg Potassium: 226mg Phosphorus: 75mg

Arugula Eggs with Chili Peppers

Preparation Time: 7 minutes

Cooking Time: 10 minutes

Servings: 4

Ingredients:

- 2 cups arugula, chopped
- 3 eggs, beaten
- ½ chili pepper, chopped
- 1 tablespoon butter
- 1 oz Parmesan, grated

Directions:

1. Toss butter in the skillet and melt it.
2. Add arugula and sauté it over medium heat for 5 minutes. Stir it from time to time.
3. Meanwhile, mix up together Parmesan, chili pepper, and eggs.
4. Pour the egg mixture over the arugula and scramble well.
5. Cook for 5 minutes more over medium heat.

Nutrition: Calories: 218 Fat: 15g Carbs: 2.8g Protein: 17g Sodium: 656mg Potassium: 243mg Phosphorus: 310mg

Eggplant Chicken Sandwich

Preparation Time: 10 minutes

Cooking Time: 15 minutes

Servings: 2

Ingredients:

- 1 eggplant, trimmed
- 10 oz chicken fillet
- 1 teaspoon Plain yogurt
- ½ teaspoon minced garlic
- 1 tablespoon fresh cilantro, chopped
- 2 lettuce leaves
- 1 teaspoon olive oil
- ½ teaspoon salt
- ½ teaspoon chili pepper
- 1 teaspoon butter

Directions:

1. Slice the eggplant lengthwise into 4 slices.
2. Rub the eggplant slices with minced garlic and brush with olive oil.
3. Grill the eggplant slices on the preheated to 375F grill for 3 minutes from each side.
4. Meanwhile, rub the chicken fillet with salt and chili pepper.
5. Place it in the skillet and add butter.

6. Roast the chicken for 6 minutes from each side over medium-high heat.

7. Cool the cooked eggplants gently and spread one side of them with Plain yogurt.

8. Add lettuce leaves and chopped fresh cilantro.

9. After this, slice the cooked chicken fillet and add over the lettuce.

10. Cover it with the remaining sliced eggplant to get the sandwich shape. Pin the sandwich with the toothpick if needed.

Nutrition: Calories: 276 Fat: 11g Carbs: 41g Protein: 13.8g Sodium: 775mg Potassium: 532mg Phosphorus: 187mg

Apple Pumpkin Muffins

Preparation time: 15 minutes

Cooking time: 20 minutes

Servings: 12

Ingredients

- 1 cup all-purpose flour
- 1 cup wheat bran
- 2 teaspoons phosphorus powder
- 1 cup pumpkin purée
- ¼ cup honey
- ¼ cup olive oil
- 1 egg
- 1 teaspoon vanilla extract
- ½ cup cored diced apple

Directions

1. Preheat the oven to 400°f.
2. Line 12 muffin cups with paper liners.
3. Stir together the flour, wheat bran, and baking powder, mix this in a medium bowl.
4. In a small bowl, whisk together the pumpkin, honey, olive oil, egg, and vanilla.
5. Stir the pumpkin mixture into the flour mixture until just combined.
6. Stir in the diced apple.

7. Spoon the batter in the muffin cups.

8. Bake for about 20 minutes, or until a toothpick inserted in the center of a muffin comes out clean.

Nutrition per serving: (1 muffin): calories: 125; total fat: 5g; saturated fat: 1g; cholesterol: 18mg; sodium: 8mg; carbohydrates: 20g; fiber: 3g; phosphorus: 120mg; potassium: 177mg; protein: 2g

LUNCH

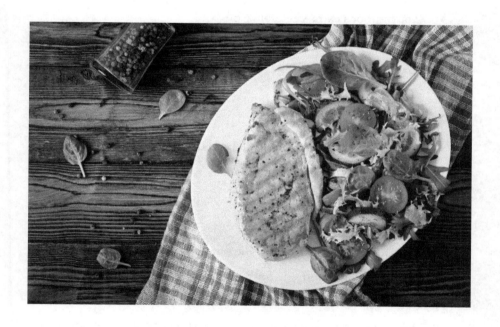

Ginger Shrimp with Snow Peas

Preparation Time: 20 minutes

Cooking Time: 12 minutes

Servings: 4

Ingredients:

- 2 tablespoons extra-virgin olive oil
- 1 tablespoon minced peeled fresh ginger
- 2 cups snow peas
- 1½ cups frozen baby peas
- 3 tablespoons water
- 1-pound medium shrimp, shelled and deveined
- 2 tablespoons low-sodium soy sauce
- 1/8 teaspoon freshly ground black pepper

Directions:

1. In a large wok or skillet, heat the olive oil over medium heat.
2. Add the ginger and stir-fry for 1 to 2 minutes, until the ginger is fragrant.
3. Add the snow peas and stir-fry for 2 to 3 minutes, until they are tender-crisp.
4. Add the baby peas and the water and stir. Cover the wok and steam for 2 to 3 minutes or until the vegetables are tender.
5. Stir in the shrimp and stir-fry for 3 to 4 minutes, or until the shrimp have curled and turned pink.
6. Add the soy sauce and pepper; stir and serve.

7. Ingredient Tip: Snow peas can have a tough string along one side that won't soften very well during the stir-fry process. Just pinch the curly end of the pod and pull to remove it. Discard the string.

Nutrition: Calories: 237; Total fat: 7g; Saturated fat: 1g; Sodium: 469mg; Phosphorus: 350mg; Potassium: 504mg; Carbohydrates: 12g; Fiber: 4g; Protein: 32g; Sugar: 5g

Roasted Cod with Plums

Preparation Time: 10 minutes

Cooking Time: 20 minutes

Servings: 4

Ingredients:

- 6 red plums, halved and pitted
- 1½ pounds cod fillets
- 3 tablespoons extra-virgin olive oil
- 2 tablespoons freshly squeezed lemon juice
- ½ teaspoon dried thyme leaves
- 1/8 teaspoon salt
- 1/8 teaspoon freshly ground black pepper
- ¾ cup plain whole-almond milk yogurt, for serving

Directions:

1. Preheat the oven to 375°F. Line a baking sheet with parchment paper.

2. Arrange the plums, cut-side up, along with the fish on the prepared baking sheet. Drizzle with the olive oil and lemon juice and sprinkle with the thyme, salt, and pepper.

3. Roast for 15 to 20 minutes or until the fish flakes when tested with a fork and the plums are tender.

4. Serve with the yogurt.

5. Ingredient Tip: There's no need to measure out exactly 2 tablespoons of lemon juice. A standard-size lemon has approximately 2 tablespoons juice in it. Simply squeeze all the juice from the lemon, being careful to avoid squeezing in the seeds.

Nutrition: Calories: 230; Total fat: 9g; Saturated fat: 2g; Sodium: 154mg; Phosphorus: 197mg; Potassium: 437mg; Carbohydrates: 10g; Fiber: 1g; Protein: 27g; Sugar: 8g

Lemon Chicken

Preparation Time: 20 minutes

Cooking Time: 24 minutes

Servings: 4

Ingredients:

- 2 lemons
- 12 ounces' boneless skinless chicken breasts, cubed
- 2 tablespoons extra-virgin olive oil
- 1/8 teaspoon salt
- 1/8 teaspoon freshly ground black pepper
- ½ large onion, chopped
- 1 cup 2-inch green bean pieces
- 1 cup 2-inch asparagus pieces

Directions:

1. Zest one of the lemons and place the zest into a medium bowl. Juice that lemon and add the juice to the bowl. Slice the remaining lemon, remove the seeds, and set aside.

2. In the bowl with the lemon juice, place the cubed chicken and set aside for 10 minutes to marinate.

3. When ready to cook, in a large skillet, heat the olive oil over medium heat.

4. Using a slotted spoon, remove the chicken from the lemon juice, reserving the lemon juice mixture. Add the chicken to the pan and cook for 3 to 4 minutes, stirring, until the chicken is lightly browned.

It doesn't have to be completely cooked. Transfer the chicken to a clean plate and sprinkle with the salt and pepper.

5. Add the sliced lemon to the skillet and cook for 3 minutes on each side, turning once, until it is slightly caramelized. Transfer to the plate with the chicken.

6. Add the onion to the skillet and cook for 3 to 4 minutes, until the onion is tender-crisp, stirring to loosen the chicken drippings from the skillet.

7. Add the green beans and sauté for 2 minutes. Add the asparagus and sauté for 1 minute.

8. Return the chicken to the skillet and add the reserved lemon juice. Simmer for 4 to 6 minutes or until the chicken is thoroughly cooked to 165°F, the vegetables are tender, and the sauce has slightly thickened.

9. Add the caramelized lemon slices to the skillet and cook for 1 to 2 minutes, stirring, until hot. Serve.

Nutrition: Calories: 207; Total fat: 9g; Saturated fat: 1g; Sodium: 121mg; Phosphorus: 245mg; Potassium: 593mg; Carbohydrates: 11g; Fiber: 4g; Protein: 22g; Sugar: 5g

Vegetable Casserole

Preparation Time: 15 minutes

Cooking Time: 15 minutes

Servings: 8

Ingredients:

- 1 teaspoon olive oil
- 1 sweet onion, chopped
- 1 teaspoon garlic, minced
- 2 zucchinis, chopped
- 1 red bell pepper, diced
- 2 carrots, chopped
- 2 cups low-sodium vegetable stock
- 2 large Red bell peppers, chopped
- 2 cups broccoli florets
- 1 teaspoon ground coriander
- ½ teaspoon ground comminutes
- Black pepper

Directions:

1. Heat the olive oil into a big pan over medium-high heat.
2. Add onion and garlic. Softly cook for about 3 minutes until softened.
3. Include the zucchini, carrots, bell pepper and softly cook for 5-6 minutes.
4. Pour the vegetable stock, Red bell peppers, broccoli, coriander, cumin, pepper and stir well.

5. Softly cook for about 5 minutes over medium-high heat until the vegetables are tender.

6. Serve hot and enjoy!

Nutrition: Calories 47 Fat 1 g Cholesterol 0 g Carbohydrates 8 g Sugar 6 g Fiber 2 g Protein 2 g Sodium 104 mg Calcium 36 mg Phosphorus 52 mg Potassium 298 mg

DINNER

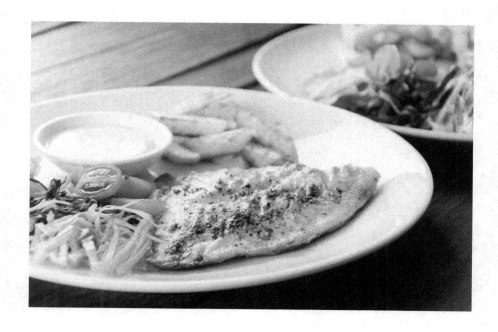

Chicken and Apple Curry

Preparation Time: 10 minutes

Cooking Time: 1 hour and 11 minutes

Servings: 8

Ingredients:

- 8 boneless skinless chicken breasts
- 1/4 teaspoon black pepper
- 2 medium apples, peeled, cored, and chopped
- 2 small onions, chopped
- 1 garlic clove, minced
- 3 tablespoons butter
- 1 tablespoon curry powder
- 1/2 tablespoon dried basil
- 3 tablespoons flour
- 1 cup chicken broth
- 1 cup of rice almond milk

Directions:

1. Preheat oven to 350°F.
2. Set the chicken breasts in a baking pan and sprinkle black pepper over it.
3. Place a suitably-sized saucepan over medium heat and add butter to melt.
4. Add onion, garlic, and apple, then sauté until soft.

5. Stir in basil and curry powder, and then cook for 1 minute.

6. Add flour and continue mixing for 1 minute.

7. Stir in rice almond milk and chicken broth, then stir cook for 5 minutes.

8. Pour this sauce over the chicken breasts in the baking pan.

9. Bake the chicken for 60 minutes then serve.

Nutrition: Calories: 232 kcal Total Fat: 8 g Saturated Fat: 0 g Cholesterol: 85 mg Sodium: 118 mg Total Carbs: 11 g

London Broil

Preparation Time: 10 minutes

Cooking Time: 5 minutes

Servings: 4

Ingredients:

- 2 pounds flank steak
- 1/4 teaspoon meat tenderizer
- 1 tablespoon sugar
- 2 tablespoons lemon juice
- 2 tablespoons soy sauce
- 1 tablespoon honey
- 1 teaspoon herb seasoning blend

Directions:

1. Pound the meat with a mallet then place it in a shallow dish.
2. Sprinkle meat tenderizer over the meat.
3. Whisk rest of the ingredients and spread this marinade over the meat.
4. Marinate the meat for 4 hours in the refrigerator.
5. Bake the meat for 5 minutes per side at 350°F.
6. Slice and serve.

Nutrition: Calories: 184 kcal Total Fat: 8 g   Saturated Fat: 0 g Cholesterol: 43 mg Sodium: 208 mg Total Carbs: 3 g

Sirloin with Squash and Pineapple

Preparation Time: 10 minutes

Cooking Time: 9 minutes

Servings: 2

Ingredients:

- 8 ounces canned pineapple slices
- 2 garlic cloves, minced
- 2 teaspoons ginger root, minced
- 3 teaspoons olive oil
- 1 pound sirloin tips
- 1 medium zucchini, diced
- 1 medium yellow squash, diced
- 1/2 medium red onion, diced

Directions:

1. Mix pineapple juice with 1 teaspoon olive oil, ginger, and garlic in a Ziplock bag.
2. Add sirloin tips to the pineapple juice marinade and seal the bag.
3. Place the bag in the refrigerator overnight.
4. Preheat oven to 450°F.
5. Layer 2 sheet pans with foil and grease it with 1 teaspoon olive oil.

6. Spread the squash, onion, and pineapple rings in the prepared pans.

7. Bake them for 5 minutes then transfer to the serving plate.

8. Place the marinated sirloin tips on a baking sheet and bake for 4 minutes in the oven.

9. Transfer the sirloin tips to the roasted vegetables.

10. Serve.

Nutrition: Calories: 264 kcal Total Fat: 12 g Saturated Fat: 0 g Cholesterol: 74 mg Sodium: 150 mg Total Carbs: 14 g

Falafel

Preparation Time: 10 minutes

Cooking time: 6 minutes

Servings: 4 servings

Ingredients:

- 1 cup chickpeas, soaked, cooked
- 1/3 cup white onion, diced
- 3 garlic cloves, chopped
- 3 tablespoons fresh parsley, chopped
- 1 tablespoon chickpea flour
- ½ teaspoon salt
- ½ teaspoon ground cumin
- ¾ teaspoon ground coriander
- ½ teaspoon chili flakes
- ½ teaspoon cayenne pepper
- ½ teaspoon ground cardamom
- 3 tablespoons olive oil

Directions:

1. Blend chickpeas, onion, garlic cloves, parsley, chickpea flour, salt, ground cumin, ground coriander, chili flakes, cayenne pepper ground cardamom.

2. When the chickpea mixture is homogenous and smooth transfer it in the mixing bowl.

3. Make the medium balls from the chickpea mixture.

4. Pour olive oil in the skillet and heat it.

5. Fry the chickpea balls for 2 minutes from each side over the medium heat.

6. The cooked falafel should have a light brown color.

7. Dry the falafel with a paper towel if needed.

Nutrition: calories 283, fat 13.7, fiber 9.2, carbs 32.6, protein 10.1

MAIN

Spicy Marble Eggs

Preparation Time: 15 minutes

Cooking Time: 2 hours

Servings: 12

Ingredients:

- 6 medium-boiled eggs, unpeeled, cooled
- For the Marinade
- 2 oolong black tea bags
- 3 Tbsp. brown sugar
- 1 thumb-sized fresh ginger, unpeeled, crushed
- 3 dried star anise, whole
- 2 dried bay leaves
- 3 Tbsp. light soy sauce
- 4 Tbsp. dark soy sauce
- 4 cups of water
- 1 dried cinnamon stick, whole
- 1 tsp. salt
- 1 tsp. dried Szechuan peppercorns

Directions:

1. Using the back of a metal spoon, crack eggshells in places to create a spider web effect. Do not peel. Set aside until needed.
2. Pour marinade into large Dutch oven set over high heat. Put lid partially on. Bring water to a rolling boil, about 5 minutes. Turn off heat.
3. Secure lid. Steep ingredients for 10 minutes.
4. Using a slotted spoon, fish out and discard solids. Cool marinade completely to room proceeding.
5. Place eggs into an airtight non-reactive container just small enough to snugly fit all these in.
6. Pour in marinade. Eggs should be completely submerged in liquid. Discard leftover marinade, if any. Line container rim with generous layers of saran wrap. Secure container lid.
7. Chill eggs for 24 hours before using.
8. Extract eggs and drain each piece well before using, but keep the rest submerged in the marinade.

Nutrition: Calories: 75 kcal Protein: 4.05 g Fat: 4.36 g Carbohydrates: 4.83 g

Nutty Oats Pudding

Preparation Time: 5 minutes

Cooking Time: 0 minutes

Servings: 3 -5

Ingredients:

- ¼ cup rolled oats
- 1 tablespoon yogurt, fat-free
- 1 ½ tablespoon natural peanut butter
- ¼ cup dry almond milk
- 1 teaspoon peanuts, finely chopped
- ½ cup of water

Directions:

1. Using a microwaveable-safe bowl, put together peanut butter and dry almond milk. Whisk well. Add in water to achieve a smooth consistency. Add in oats.

2. Cover bowl with plastic wrap. Create a small hole for the steam to escape.

3. Place inside the microwave oven for 1 minute on high powder.

4. Continue heating, this time on medium power for 90 seconds. Let sit for 5 minutes.

5. To serve, spoon an equal amount of cereals in a bowl top with peanuts and yogurt.

Nutrition: Calories: 70 kcal Protein: 4.25 g Fat: 3.83 g Carbohydrates: 6.78 g

Almond Pancakes with Coconut Flakes

Preparation: Time: 5 minutes

Cooking Time: 10 minutes

Servings: 6

Ingredients:

- 1 overripe banana, mashed
- 2 eggs, yolks, and whites separated
- ½ cup unsweetened applesauce
- 1 cup almond flour, finely milled
- ¼ cup of water
- ¼ tsp. coconut oil
- Garnish
- 2 Tbsp. blanched almond flakes
- Dash of cinnamon powder
- ¼ cup coconut flakes, sweetened
- Pinch of sea salt
- Pure maple syrup, use sparingly

Directions:

1. Whisk egg whites until soft peaks form.
2. Except for egg whites and coconut oil, combine remaining ingredients in another bowl. Mix until batter comes together.
3. Gently fold in egg whites. Make sure that you don't over mix, or the pancake will become dense and chewy.
4. Pour oil into a nonstick skillet set over medium heat.

5. Wait for the oil to heat up before dropping in approximately ½ cup of batter. Cook until each side are set, and bubbles form in the center. Turn on the other side then cook for another 2 minutes.

6. Transfer flapjacks to a plate. Repeat step until all batter is cooked. Pour in more oil into the skillet only if needed. This recipe should yield between 4 to 6 medium-sized pancakes.

7. Stack pancakes. Pour the desired amount of pure maple syrup on top. Garnish each stack with cinnamon-flavored almond-coconut flakes just before serving.

8. For the garnish, set the oven to 350°F for at least 10 minutes before use. Line a baking sheet with parchment paper. Set aside.

9. Mix almond and coconut flakes together in a bowl. Spread mixture evenly on a prepared baking sheet.

10. Bake for 7 to 10 minutes until flakes turn golden brown. Stir almond and coconut flakes once midway through roasting to prevent over-browning.

11. Remove the baking sheet from the oven. Cool almond and coconut flakes for at least 10 minutes before sprinkling in cinnamon powder and salt. Toss to combine. Set aside.

Nutrition: Calories: 62 kcal Protein: 2.24 g Fat: 4.01 g Carbohydrates: 4.46 g

Banana Pancakes

Preparation Time: 5 minutes

Cooking Time: 15 minutes

Servings: 2

Ingredients:

- 2 Eggs
- 1 Egg White
- 1 Banana, Ripe
- 1 Cup Rolled Oats
- 2 Teaspoons Ground Cinnamon
- 1 Tablespoon Coconut Oil, Divided
- 1 Teaspoon Vanilla Extract, Pure
- ½ Teaspoon Sea Salt

Directions:

1. Get out a food processor, grinding your oats until they make a coarse flour.

2. Add your cinnamon, egg whites, eggs, banana, vanilla, and salt. Blend until it forms a smooth batter, and then heat a small skillet over medium heat. Heat a half a tablespoon of coconut oil, and then pour your batter in. Cook for two minutes per side, and continue until all of your batter has been used.

Nutrition: Calories: 306 Protein: 15 Grams Fat: 15 Grams Carbs: 17 Grams

SIDES

Thai-Style Eggplant Dip

Preparation Time: 10 minutes

Cooking Time: 30 minutes

Servings: 4

Ingredients:

- 1 pound Thai eggplant (or Japanese or Chinese eggplant)
- 2 tablespoons rice vinegar
- 2 teaspoons sugar
- 1 teaspoon low-sodium soy sauce
- 1 jalapeño pepper
- 2 garlic cloves
- ¼ cup chopped basil
- Cut vegetables for serving

Directions:

1. Preheat the oven to 475°F
2. Pierce the eggplant in several places with a skewer or knife. Place on a rimmed baking sheet and cook until soft, about 30 minutes.
3. Let cool, cut in half, and scoop out the flesh of the eggplant into a blender.
4. Add the rice vinegar, sugar, soy sauce, jalapeño, garlic, and basil to the blender. Process until smooth. Serve with cut vegetables

5. Lower sodium tip: If you need to lower your sodium further, omit the soy sauce to lower the sodium to 3mg.

Nutrition: Calories: 40; Total Fat: 0g; Saturated Fat: 0g; Cholesterol: 0mg; Carbohydrates: 10g; Fiber: 4g;Protein: 2g; Phosphorus: 34mg; Potassium: 284mg; Sodium: 47mg

Collard Salad Rolls with Peanut Dipping Sauce

Preparation Time: 10 minutes

Cooking Time: 10 minutes

Servings: 4

Ingredients:

FOR THE DIPPING SAUCE

- ¼ cup peanut butter
- 2 tablespoons honey
- Juice of 1 lime
- ¼ teaspoon red chili flakes

FOR THE SALAD ROLLS

- 4 ounces' extra-firm tofu
- 1 bunch collard greens
- 1 cup thinly sliced purple cabbage
- 1 cup bean sprouts
- 2 carrots, cut into matchsticks
- ½ cup cilantro leaves and stems

Directions:

TO MAKE THE DIPPING SAUCE

1. In a blender, combine the peanut butter, honey, lime juice, chili flakes, and process until smooth. Put 1 to 2 tablespoons of water as desired for consistency.

TO MAKE THE SALAD ROLLS

2. Using paper towels, press the excess moisture from the tofu. Cut into ½-inch-thick matchsticks.

3. Remove any tough stems from the collard greens and set aside.

4. Arrange all of the ingredients within reach. Cup one collard green leaf in your hand, and add a couple pieces of the tofu and a small amount each of the cabbage, bean sprouts, and carrots. Top with a couple cilantro sprigs, and roll into a cylinder. Place each roll, seam-side down, on a serving platter while you assemble the rest of the rolls. Serve with the dipping sauce.

5. Substitution tip: To lower the potassium, omit the cabbage and use only 1 carrot, which will drop the potassium to 208mg.

Nutrition: Calories: 174; Total Fat: 9g; Saturated Fat: 2g; Cholesterol: 0mg; Carbohydrates: 20g; Fiber: 5g;Protein: 8g; Phosphorus: 56mg; Potassium: 284mg; Sodium: 42mg

Corn Bread

Preparation Time: 10 minutes

Cooking Time: 20 minutes

Servings: 10

Ingredients:

- Cooking spray for greasing the baking dish
- Yellow cornmeal – 1 ¼ cups
- All-purpose flour – ¾ cup
- Baking soda substitute – 1 tbsp.
- Granulated sugar – ½ cup
- Eggs – 2
- Unsweetened, unfortified rice almond milk – 1 cup
- Olive oil – 2 Tbsps.

Directions:

1. Preheat the oven to 425F.
2. Lightly spray an 8-by-8-inch baking dish with cooking spray. Set aside.
3. In a medium bowl, stir together the cornmeal, flour, baking soda substitute, and sugar.
4. In a small bowl, whisk together the eggs, rice almond milk, and olive oil until blended.
5. Place the wet ingredients to the dry ingredients and stir until well combined.
6. Pour the batter into the baking dish and bake for 20 minutes or until golden and cooked through.
7. Serve warm.

Nutrition: Calories: 198 Fat: 5g Carb: 34g Phosphorus: 88mg Potassium: 94mg Sodium: 25mg Protein: 4g

SALAD

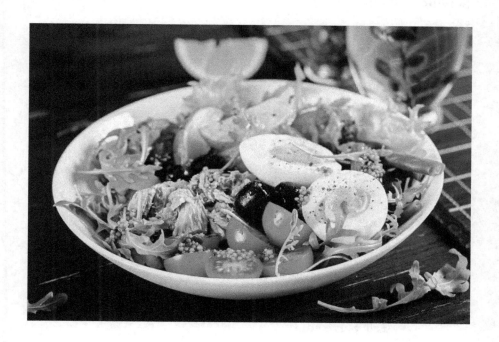

Tuna macaroni salad

Preparation time: 5 minutes

Cooking time: 25 minutes

Servings: 10 servings

Ingredients:

- 1 1/2 cups Uncooked Macaroni
- 1 170g Can of tuna in water
- 1/4 cup Mayonnaise
- 2 medium celery stalks, diced
- 1 Tbsp. Lemon Pepper Seasoning

Directions:

1. Cook the pasta and let it cool in the refrigerator.
2. Drain the tuna in a colander and rinse it with cold water.
3. Add the tuna and celery once the macaroni has cooled.
4. Stir in mayonnaise and sprinkle with lemon seasoning. Mix well. Serve cold.

Nutrition: Power: 136 g, Protein: 8.0 g, Carbohydrates: 18 g, fibbers: 0.8 g, Fat: 3.6 g, Sodium: 75 mg, Potassium: 124 mg, Phosphorus: 90 mg

Couscous salad

Preparation time: 5 minutes

Cooking time: 5 minutes

Servings: 5 servings

Ingredients:

- 3 cups of water
- 1/2 tsp. cinnamon tea
- 1/2 tsp. cumin tea
- 1 tsp. honey soup
- 2 tbsp. lemon juice
- 3 cups quick-cooking couscous
- 2 tbsp. tea of olive oil
- 1 green onion,
- Finely chopped 1 small carrot, finely diced
- 1/2 red pepper,
- Finely diced fresh coriander

Directions:

1. Stir in the water with the cinnamon, cumin, honey, and lemon juice and bring to a boil. Put the couscous in it, cover it, and remove it from the heat. To swell the couscous, stir with a fork. Add the vegetables, fresh herbs, and olive oil. It is possible to serve the salad warm or cold.

Nutrition: Energy: 190 g, Protein: 6 g, Carbohydrates: 38 g, fibbers: 2 g, Total Fat: 1 g, Sodium: 4 mg, Phosphorus: 82 mg, Potassium: 116 mg

POULTRY

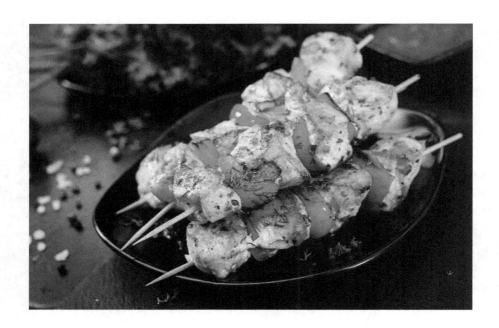

Herbs and Lemony Roasted Chicken

Preparation Time: 15 Minutes

Cooking Time: 1 Hour and 30 Minutes

Servings: 8

Ingredients:

- 1/2 teaspoon ground black pepper
- 1/2 teaspoon mustard powder
- 1/2 teaspoon salt
- 1 3-lb whole chicken
- 1 teaspoon garlic powder
- 2 lemons
- 2 tablespoons. olive oil
- 2 teaspoons. Italian seasoning

Directions:

1. In a small bowl, mix black pepper, garlic powder, mustard powder, and salt.

2. Rinse chicken well and slice off giblets.

3. In a greased 9 x 13 baking dish, place chicken on it. Add 11/2 teaspoon of seasoning made earlier inside the chicken and rub the remaining seasoning around the chicken.

4. In a small bowl, mix olive oil and juice from 2 lemons. Drizzle over chicken.

5. Bake chicken in an oven preheated at 3500 F until juices run clear, for around 11/2 hour. Occasionally, baste the chicken with its juices.

Nutrition: Calories per Serving 190, Carbohydrates 2g, protein 35g, fats 9g, phosphorus 341mg, potassium 439mg, sodium 328mg

Ground Chicken and Peas Curry

Preparation Time: 15 Minutes

Cooking Time: 6 to 10 Minutes

Servings: 3-4

Ingredients:

For Marinade:

- 3 tablespoons essential olive oil
- 2 bay leaves
- 2 onions, ground to some paste
- 1/2 tablespoon garlic paste
- 1/2 tablespoon ginger paste
- 2 Red bell peppers, chopped finely
- 1 tablespoon ground cumin
- 1 tablespoon ground coriander
- 1 teaspoon ground turmeric
- 1 teaspoon red chili powder
- Salt, to taste
- 1-pound lean ground chicken
- 2 cups frozen peas
- 11/2 cups water
- 1-2 teaspoons garam masala powder

Directions:

1. In a deep skillet, heat oil on medium heat.
2. Add bay leaves and sauté for approximately half a minute.
3. Add onion paste and sauté for approximately 3-4 minutes.
4. Add garlic and ginger paste and sauté for around 1-11/2 minutes.
5. Add Red bell peppers and spices, and cook, stirring occasionally for about 3-4 minutes.
6. Stir in chicken and cook for about 4-5 minutes.
7. Stir in peas and water and bring to a boil on high heat.
8. Reduce the heat to low and simmer approximately 5-8 minutes or till desired doneness.
9. Stir in garam masala and remove from heat.
10. Serve hot.

Nutrition: Calories 450, Fat 10g, Carbohydrates 19g, Fiber 6g, Protein 38g

White Bean, Chicken & Apple Cider Chili

Preparation Time: 15 minutes

Cooking Time: 7 to 8 hours

Servings: 4

Ingredients:

- 3 cups chopped cooked chicken (see Basic "Rotisserie" Chicken)
- 2 (15-ounce) cans white navy beans, rinsed well and drained
- 1 medium onion, chopped
- 1 (15-ounce) can diced bell pepper
- 3 cups Chicken Bone Broth or store-bought chicken broth
- 1 cup apple cider
- 2 bay leaves
- 1 tablespoon extra-virgin oil
- 2 teaspoons garlic powder
- 1 teaspoon chili powder
- 1 teaspoon salt
- ½ teaspoon ground cumin
- ¼ teaspoon ground cinnamon
- Pinch cayenne pepper
- Freshly ground black pepper
- ¼ cup apple cider vinegar

Directions:

1. In your slow cooker, combine the chicken, beans, onion, bell pepper, broth, cider, bay leaves, oil, garlic powder, chili powder, salt, cumin, cinnamon cayenne, and season with black pepper.

2. Cover the cooker and set to low. Cook for 7 to 8 hours.

3. Remove and discard the bay leaves. Stir in the apple cider vinegar until well blended and serve.

Nutrition: Calories: 469 Total Fat: 8g Total Carbs: 46g Sugar: 13g Fiber: 9g Protein: 51g Sodium: 147mg

SEAFOOD

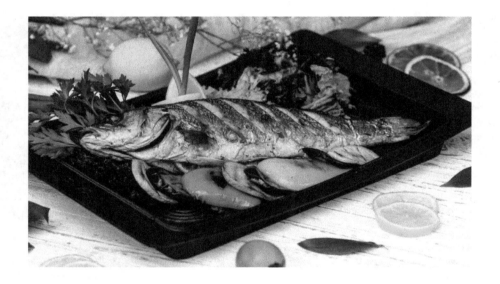

Smoked Salmon and Radishes

Preparation Time: 10 minutes

CookingTime:10minutes

Servings: 8

Ingredients:

- ½ c. drained and chopped capers
- 1 lb. skinless, de-boned and flaked smoked salmon
- 4 chopped radishes
- 3 tbsps. Chopped chives
- 3 tbsps. Prepared beet horseradish
- 2 tsps. Grated lemon zest
- 1/3 c. roughly chopped red onion

Directions:

1. In a bowl, combine the salmon while using the beet horseradish, lemon zest, radish, capers, onions and chives, toss and serve cold.

2. Enjoy!

Nutrition: Calories: 254, Fat: 2 g, Carbs: 7 g, Protein: 7 g, Sugars: 1.4 g, Sodium: 660 mg

Parmesan Baked Fish

Preparation Time: 10 minutes

CookingTime:10minutes

Servings: 4

Ingredients:

- ½ tsp. Worcestershire sauce

- 1/3 c. mayonnaise

- 3 tbsps. Freshly grated parmesan cheese

- 4 oz. cod fish fillets

- 1 tbsp. snipped fresh chives

Directions:

1. Preheat oven to 450°C.

2. Rinse fish and pat dry with paper towels; spray an 8x8x2 baking dish with non-stick pan spray, set aside.

3. In small bowl stir mayo, grated cheese, chives, and Worcestershire sauce; spread mixture over fish fillets.

4. Bake, uncovered, 12-15 minutes or until fish flakes easily with a fork

Nutrition: Calories: 850.5, Fat: 24.8g, Carbs: 44.5 g, Protein: 104.6 g, Sugars: 0.6 g, Sodium: 307.7 mg

Shrimp and Mango Mix

Preparation Time: 10 minutes

CookingTime:10minutes

Servings: 4

Ingredients:

- 3 tbsps. Finely chopped parsley
- 3 tbsps. Coconut sugar
- 1 lb. peeled, deveined and cooked shrimp
- 3 tbsps. Balsamic vinegar
- 3 peeled and cubed mangos

Directions:

1. In a bowl, mix vinegar with sugar and mayo and whisk.
2. In another bowl, combine the mango with the parsley and shrimp, add the mayo mix, toss and serve.
3. Enjoy!

Nutrition: Calories: 204, Fat: 3 g, Carbs: 8 g, Protein: 8 g, Sugars: 12.6 g, Sodium: 273.4 mg

Roasted hake

Preparation Time: 20 minutes

CookingTime:30minutes

Servings: 4

Ingredients:

- ½ c. tomato sauce
- 2 sliced Red bell peppers
- Fresh parsley
- ½ c. grated cheese
- 4 lbs. deboned hake fish
- 1 tbsp. olive oil
- Salt.

Directions:

1. Season the fish with salt. Pan-fry the fish until half-done.
2. Shape foil into containers according to the number of fish pieces.
3. Pour tomato sauce into each foil dish; arrange the fish, then the tomato slices, again add tomato sauce and sprinkle with grated cheese.
4. Bake in the oven at 400 F until there is a golden crust.
5. Serve with fresh parsley.

Nutrition: Calories: 421, Fat: 48.7 g, Carbs: 2.4 g, Protein: 17.4 g, Sugars: 0.5 g, Sodium: 94.6 mg

MEAT

Pork Loins with Leeks

Preparation Time: 10 minutes

Cooking Time: 35 minutes

Servings: 2

Ingredients:

- 1 sliced leek
- 1 tablespoon mustard seeds
- 6-ounce pork tenderloin
- 1 tablespoon cumin seeds
- 1 tablespoon dry mustard
- 1 tablespoon extra-virgin oil

Directions:

1. Preheat the broiler to medium-high heat. In a dry skillet, heat mustard and cumin seeds until they start to pop (3-5 minutes). Grind seeds using a pestle and mortar or blender and then mix in the dry mustard.

2. Massage the pork on all sides using the mustard blend and add to a baking tray to broil for 25-30 minutes or until cooked through. Turn once halfway through.
3. Remove and place to one side, then heat-up the oil in a pan on medium heat and add the leeks for 5-6 minutes or until soft. Serve the pork tenderloin on a bed of leeks and enjoy it!

Nutrition: Calories 139 Fat 5g Carbs 2g Phosphorus 278mg Potassium 45mg Sodium 47mg Protein 18g

SNACK

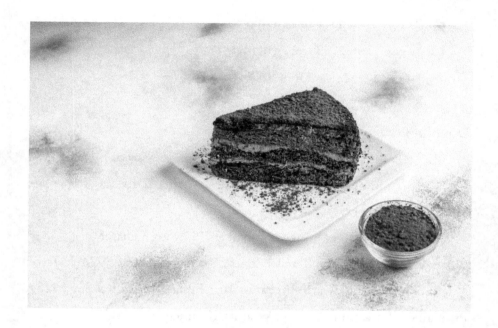

Mango Chiller

Preparation time: 5 minutes

Cooking time: 5 minutes

Servings: 4 (½ cup per serving)

Ingredients:

- 2 cups frozen mango chunks
- ½ cup plain 2% Greek yogurt
- ¼ cup 1% almond milk
- 2 teaspoons honey (optional

Direction:

1. Mix the mango and yogurt in a food processor or blender. Add the almond milk, a bit at a time, to get it to soft ice cream consistency.

2. Taste, and add honey if you like. Enjoy immediately.

Nutrition: Calories: 85; Total Fat: 1g; Saturated Fat: 1g; Cholesterol: 4mg; Sodium: 17mg; Carbohydrates: 16g; Fiber: 1g; Added Sugars: 3g; Protein: 4g; Potassium: 197mg; Vitamin K: 3mcg

Blueberry-Ricotta Swirl

Preparation time: 5 minutes

Cooking time: 5 minutes

Servings: 2

Ingredients:

- ½ cup fresh or frozen blueberries
- ½ cup part-skim ricotta cheese
- 1 teaspoon sugar
- ½ teaspoon lemon zest (optional)

Directions:

1. If using frozen blueberries, warm them in a saucepan over medium heat until they are thawed but not hot.
2. Meanwhile, mix the sugar with the ricotta in a medium bowl.
3. Mix the blueberries into the ricotta, leaving a few out. Taste, and add more sugar if desired. Top with the remaining blueberries and lemon zest (if using).

Nutrition: Calories: 113; Total Fat: 5g; Saturated Fat: 3g; Cholesterol: 19mg; Sodium: 62mg; Carbohydrates: 10g; Fiber: 1g; Added Sugars: 2g; Protein: 7g; Potassium: 98mg; Vitamin K: 7mcg

Roasted Broccoli and Cauliflower

Preparation Time: 7 minutes

Cooking Time: 23 minutes

Serving: 6

Ingredients:

- 2 cups broccoli florets
- 2 cups cauliflower florets
- 2 tablespoons olive oil
- 1 tablespoon freshly squeezed lemon juice
- 2 teaspoons Dijon mustard
- ¼ teaspoon garlic powder
- Pinch salt
- 1/8 teaspoon freshly ground black pepper

Direction

1. Preheat the oven to 425°F.
2. On a baking sheet with a lip, combine the broccoli and cauliflower florets in one even layer.
3. In a small bowl, combine the olive oil, lemon juice, mustard, garlic powder, salt, and pepper until well blended and drizzle the mixture over the vegetables. Toss to coat and spread the vegetables out in a single layer again.
4. Roast for 22 minutes. Serve immediately.

Nutrition: 63   Calories74mg   Sodium39mg   Phosphorus216mg
Potassium2g Protein

Herbed Garlic Cauliflower Mash

Preparation Time: 10 minutes

Cooking Time: 20 minutes

Serving: 6

Ingredients:

- 4 cups cauliflower florets
- 4 garlic cloves, peeled
- 4 ounces cream cheese, softened
- ¼ cup unsweetened almond milk
- 2 tablespoons unsalted butter
- Pinch salt
- 2 tablespoons minced fresh chives
- 2 tablespoons chopped flat-leaf parsley
- 1 tablespoon fresh thyme leaves

Direction

1. Boil water at high heat. Add the cauliflower and garlic and cook, stirring occasionally, until the cauliflower is tender, about 8 to 10 minutes.

2. Drain the cauliflower and garlic into a colander in the sink and shake the colander well to remove excess water.

3. Using a paper towel, blot the vegetables to remove any remaining water. Return the florets to the pot and place over low heat for 1 minute to remove as much water as possible.

4. Mash the florets and garlic with a potato masher until smooth.

5. Beat in the cream cheese, almond milk, butter, salt, chives, parsley, and thyme with a spoon. Serve.

Nutrition: 124 Calories115mg Sodium59mg Phosphorus266mg Potassium 3g Protein

Buffalo chicken dip

Preparation time: 10 minutes

Cooking time: 3 hours

Servings: 4

Ingredients

- 4-ounce cream cheese
- 1/2 cup bottled roasted red peppers
- 1 cup reduced-fat sour cream
- 4 teaspoon hot pepper sauce
- 2 cups cooked, shredded chicken

Directions

1. Blend half cup of drained red peppers in a food processor until smooth.
2. Now, thoroughly mix cream cheese, and sour cream with the pureed peppers in a bowl.
3. Stir in shredded chicken and hot sauce then transfer the mixture to a slow cooker.
4. Cook for 3 hours on low heat.
5. Serve warm with celery, carrots, cauliflower, and cucumber.

Nutrition: calories 73. Protein 5 g. Carbohydrates 2 g. Fat 5 g. Cholesterol 25 mg. Sodium 66 mg. Potassium 81 mg. Phosphorus 47 mg. Calcium 31 mg. Fiber 0 g.

SOUP

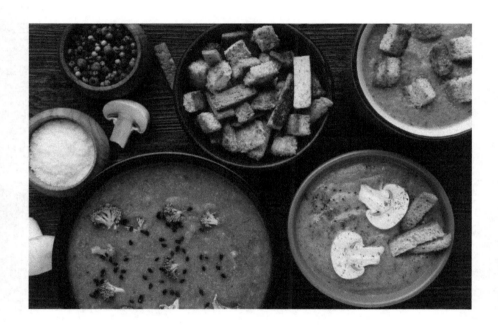

Creamy Tuna Salad

Preparation Time: 10 minutes

Cooking Time: 5 minutes

Servings: 4

Ingredients:

- oz. can tuna, drained and flaked
- 1 1/2 tsp garlic powder
- 1 tbsp. dill, chopped
- 1 tsp curry powder
- 2 tbsp. fresh lemon juice
- 1/2 cup onion, chopped
- 1/2 cup celery, chopped
- 1/4 cup parmesan cheese, grated
- /4 cup mayonnaise

Directions:

1. Add all ingredients into the large bowl and mix until well combined.
2. Serve and enjoy.

Nutrition: Calories 224 Fat 15.5 g Carbohydrates 14.1 g Sugar 4.2 g Protein 8 g Cholesterol 20 mg Phosphorus: 110mg Potassium: 117mg Sodium: 75mg

Creamy Mushroom Soup

Preparation Time: 10 minutes

Cooking Time: 15 minutes

Servings: 6

Ingredients:

- 1 lb. mushrooms, sliced
- 1/2 cup heavy cream
- 4 cups chicken broth
- 1 tbsp. sage, chopped
- 1/4 cup butter
- Pepper
- Salt

Directions:

1. Melt butter in a large pot over medium heat.
2. Add sage and saute for 1 minute.
3. Add mushrooms and cook for 3-5 minutes or until lightly browned.
4. Add broth and stir well and simmer for 5 minutes.
5. Puree the soup using an immersion blender until smooth.
6. Add heavy cream and stir well. Season soup with pepper and salt.
7. Serve hot and enjoy.

Nutrition: Calories 145 Fat 12.5 g Carbohydrates 3.6 g Sugar 1.8 g Protein 5.9 g Cholesterol 34 mg Phosphorus: 140mg Potassium: 127mg Sodium: 75mg

Pork Soup

Preparation Time: 10 minutes

Cooking Time: 4 hours 15 minutes

Servings: 8

Ingredients:

- 2 lbs. country pork ribs, boneless and cut into 1-inch pieces
- 2 cups cauliflower rice
- 1 1/2 tbsp. fresh oregano, chopped
- 1 cup of water
- 2 cups Red bell peppers, chopped
- 1 cup chicken stock
- 1/2 cup dry white wine
- 1 onion, chopped
- 3 garlic cloves, chopped
- 1 tbsp. olive oil
- Pepper
- Salt

Directions:

1. Heat oil in a saucepan over medium heat.
2. Season pork with pepper and salt. Add pork into the saucepan and cook until lightly brown from all the sides.
3. Add onion and garlic and saute for 2 minutes.
4. Add Red bell peppers, water, stock, and white wine and stir well. Bring to boil.

5. Pour saucepan mixture into the slow cooker.

6. Cover and cook on high for 4 hours.

7. Add cauliflower rice and oregano in the last 20 minutes of cooking.

8. Stir well and serve.

Nutrition: Calories 263 Fat 15.1 g Carbohydrates 5.8 g Sugar 2.6 g Protein 23.4 g Cholesterol 85 mg Phosphorus: 130mg Potassium: 117mg Sodium: 105mg

VEGETABLES

Vegetable Biryani

Preparation Time: 10 minutes

Cooking Time: 15 minutes

Servings: 4

Ingredients:

- 2 tablespoons olive oil
- 1 onion, diced
- 4 garlic cloves, minced
- 1 tbsp. peeled and grated fresh ginger root
- 1 cup carrot, grated
- 2 cups chopped cauliflower
- 1 cup thawed frozen baby peas
- 2 teaspoons curry powder
- 1 cup low-sodium vegetable broth
- 3 cups of frozen cooked white rice

Directions:

1. Get a skillet and heat the olive oil on medium heat.
2. Add onion, garlic, and ginger root. Sauté, frequently stirring, until tender-crisp, 2 minutes.

3. Add the carrot, cauliflower, peas, and curry powder and cook for 2 minutes longer.

4. Put vegetable broth. Cover the skillet partially, and simmer on low for 6 to 7 minutes or until the vegetables are tender.

5. Meanwhile, heat the rice as directed on the package.

6. Stir the rice into the vegetable mixture and serve.

Nutrition: Calories: 378Fat 16gCarbohydrates: 53gProtein: 8gSodium: 113mgPotassium: 510mg Phosphorus: 236mg

Pesto Pasta Salad

Preparation Time: 15 minutes

Cooking Time: 15 minutes

Servings: 4

Ingredients:

- 1 cup fresh basil leaves
- ½ cup packed fresh flat-leaf parsley leaves
- ½ cup arugula, chopped
- 2 tablespoons Parmesan cheese, grated
- ¼ cup extra-virgin olive oil
- 3 tablespoons mayonnaise
- 2 tablespoons water
- 12 ounces whole-wheat rotini pasta
- 1 red bell pepper, chopped
- 1 medium yellow summer squash, sliced
- 1 cup frozen baby peas

Directions:

1. Boil water in a large pot.
2. Meanwhile, combine the basil, parsley, arugula, cheese, and olive oil in a blender or food processor. Process until the herbs are finely chopped. Add the mayonnaise and water, then process again. Set aside.
3. Prepare the pasta to the pot of boiling water; cook according to package directions, about 8 to 9 minutes. Drain well, reserving ¼ cup of the cooking liquid.

4. Combine the pesto, pasta, bell pepper, squash, and peas in a large bowl and toss gently, adding enough reserved pasta cooking liquid to make a sauce on the salad. Serve immediately or cover and chill, then serve.

5. Store covered in the refrigerator for up to 3 days.

Nutrition: Calories: 378Fat: 24gCarbohydrates: 35gProtein: 9gSodium: 163mgPotassium: 472mgPhosphorus: 213mg

Barley Blueberry Salad

Preparation Time: 15 minutes

Cooking Time: 15 minutes

Servings: 4

Ingredients:

- 1 cup quick-cooking barley
- 3 cups low-sodium vegetable broth
- 3 tablespoons extra-virgin olive oil
- 2 tablespoons freshly squeezed lemon juice
- 1 teaspoon yellow mustard
- 1 teaspoon honey
- 2 cups blueberries
- ¼ cup crumbled feta cheese

Directions:

1. Combine the barley and vegetable broth in a medium saucepan and bring to a simmer.
2. Reduce the heat to low, partially cover the pan, and simmer for 10 to 12 minutes or until the barley is tender.
3. Meanwhile, whisk together the olive oil, lemon juice, mustard, and honey in a serving bowl until blended.
4. Drain the barley if necessary and add to the bowl; toss to combine.
5. Add the blueberries, and feta and toss gently. Serve.

Nutrition: Calories: 345Fat 16gCarbohydrates: 44gProtein: 7gSodium: 259mgPotassium: 301mgPhosphorus: 152mg

Stir-Fried Gingery Veggies

Preparation Time: 10 minutes

Cooking Time: 10 minutes

Servings: 4

Ingredients:

- 1 tablespoon oil
- 3 cloves of garlic, minced
- 1 onion, chopped
- 1 thumb-size ginger, sliced
- 1 tablespoon water
- 1 large carrots, peeled and julienned and seedless
- 1 large green bell pepper, julienned and seedless
- 1 large yellow bell pepper, julienned and seedless
- 1 large red bell pepper, julienned and seedless
- 1 zucchini, julienned
- Salt and pepper to taste

Directions:

1. Heat oil in a nonstick saucepan over a high flame and sauté the garlic, onion, and ginger until fragrant.
2. Stir in the rest of the ingredients.
3. Keep on stirring for at least 5 minutes until vegetables are tender.
4. Serve and enjoy.

Nutrition: Calories 70Total Fat 4g Saturated Fat 1g Total Carbs 9gNet Carbs 7gProtein 1gSugar: 4gFiber 2gSodium 173mgPotassium 163mg

CONDIMENT, BROTH & SEASONING

Herbes De Provence

Preparation Time: 15 minutes

Cooking Time: 0 minutes

Servings: 1 cup

Ingredients:

- ½ cup dried thyme
- 3 tablespoons dried marjoram
- 3 tablespoons dried savory
- 2 tablespoons dried rosemary
- 2 teaspoons dried lavender flowers
- 1 teaspoon ground fennel

Directions:

1. Put the thyme, marjoram, savory, rosemary, lavender, and fennel in a blender and pulse a few times to combine. Store for up to 6 months.

Nutrition: Calories: 3Fat: 0gCarbohydrates: 1gPhosphorus: 2mg Potassium: 9mgSodium: 0mgProtein: 0g

Lamb and Pork Seasoning

Preparation Time: 15 minutes

Cooking Time: 0 minutes

Servings: ½ cup

Ingredients:

- ¼ cup celery seed
- 2 tablespoons dried oregano
- 2 tablespoons onion powder
- 1 tablespoon dried thyme
- 1½ teaspoons garlic powder
- 1 teaspoon crushed bay leaf
- 1 teaspoon freshly ground black pepper
- 1 teaspoon ground allspice

Directions:

1. Pulse the celery seed, oregano, onion powder, thyme, garlic powder, bay leaf, pepper, and allspice in a blender a few times. Transfer the herb mixture to a small container; then, you can store it in a cool, dry place for up to 6 months.

Nutrition: Calories: 8Fat: 0gCarbohydrates: 1gPhosphorus: 9mgPotassium: 29mgSodium: 2mg Protein: 0g

DESSERTS

Tart apple granita

Preparation time: 15 minutes, plus 4 hours freezing time

Cooking time: 0

Servings: 4

Ingredients:

- ½ cup granulated sugar
- ½ cup water
- 2 cups unsweetened apple juice
- ¼ cup freshly squeezed lemon juice

Directions:

1. In a small saucepan over medium-high heat, heat the sugar and water.

2. Bring the mixture to a boil and then reduce the heat to low and simmer for about 15 minutes or until the liquid has reduced by half.

3. Remove the pan from the heat and pour the liquid into a large shallow metal pan.

4. Let the liquid cool for about 30 minutes and then stir in the apple juice and lemon juice.

5. Place the pan in the freezer.

6. After 1 hour, run a fork through the liquid to break up any ice crystals formed. Scrape down the sides as well.

7. Place the pan back in the freezer and repeat the stirring and scraping every 20 minutes, creating slush.

8. Serve when the mixture is completely frozen and looks like crushed ice, after about 3 hours.

Nutrition: calories: 157; fat: 0g; carbohydrates: 0g; phosphorus: 10mg; potassium: 141mg; sodium: 5mg; protein

Gumdrop cookies

Preparation time: 15 minutes

Cooking time: 12 minutes

Servings: 25

Ingredients:

- ½ cup of spreadable unsalted butter
- 1 medium egg
- 1 cup of brown sugar
- 1 2/3 cups of all-purpose flour, sifted
- ¼ cup of almond milk
- 1 teaspoon vanilla
- 1 teaspoon of baking powder
- 15 large gumdrops, chopped finely

Directions:

1. Preheat the oven at 400f/195c.
2. Combine the sugar, butter and egg until creamy.
3. Add the almond milk and vanilla and stir well.
4. Combine the flour with the baking powder in a different bowl. Incorporate to the sugar, butter mixture, and stir.
5. Add the gumdrops and place the mixture in the fridge for half an hour.
6. Drop the dough with tablespoonful into a lightly greased baking or cookie sheet.
7. Bake for 10-12 minutes or until golden brown.

Nutrition: Calories: 102.17 kcal Carbohydrate: 16.5 g Protein: 0.86 g Sodium: 23.42 mg Potassium: 45 mg Phosphorus: 32.15 mg Dietary fiber: 0.13 g Fat: 4 g

DRINKS & SMOOTHIES

Grapefruit Sorbet

Preparation Time: 10 minutes

Cooking Time: 5 minutes

Servings: 6

Ingredients

- ½ cup sugar
- ¼ cup water
- 1 fresh thyme sprig
- For the sorbet
- Juice of 6 pink grapefruit
- ¼ cup thyme simple syrup

Directions:

1   In a blender, combine the grapefruit juice and ¼ cup of simple syrup, and process.

2   Transfer to an airtight container and freeze for 3 to 4 hours, until firm. Serve.

3   Substitution tip: Try this with other citrus fruits, such as mangos, lemons, or limes, for an equally delicious treat.

Nutrition: Calories 117 Fat 2.1g Carbs 18.2g Protein 22.7g Potassium (K) 296mg Sodium (Na) 81mg Phosphorous 28 mg

Blackberry Sage Cocktail

Preparation Time: 5 minutes

Cooking Time: 10 minutes

Servings: 6

Ingredients:

- Sage Simple Syrup
- 1 cup water
- 1 cup0granulated sugar
- 8 fresh sage leaves, plus more for garnish
- 1-pint fresh blackberries, muddled and strained (juices reserved)
- Juice of 1/2 a lemon
- 8 oz St. Germain Liqueur
- 16 oz vodka
- seltzer water

Directions:

1. Place water and sugar in a small saucepan.
2. Simmer until sugar dissolves for 7 to 10 minutes.
3. Remove from heat. Add sage leaves, and cover, allowing the mixture for about 2 hours.
4. Combine fresh blackberry juice, lemon juice, sage simple syrup, cocktail pitcher.
5. Mix and refrigerate covered until well chilled.
6. Serve in cocktail glasses filled with ice and garnish with fresh sage leaves and top with a splash of seltzer water.

Nutrition: Calories: 68Fat: 1gCarbs: 15gProtein: 3gSodium: 3mgPotassium: 133mgPhosphorus: 38mg